THE WEIGHT LOSS JOURNEY

A Step-by-Step Guide to Success

Steven Smith

Wisdom Publishers

ISBN: 9798372844988
Imprint: Independently published

Cover design by: Art Painter
Library of Congress Control Number: 2018675309
Printed in the United States of America

*This book is dedicated to everyone that desires
to shed weight to stay healthier*

*The only way to keep your health is to eat what you don't want,
drink what you don't like, and do what you'd rather not*

MARK TWAIN

CONTENTS

INTRODUCTION

Maintaining a healthy weight is important for overall health and well-being. Being at a healthy weight can help reduce the risk of developing serious health conditions such as obesity, type 2 diabetes, heart disease, and certain types of cancer. One of the main ways to maintain a healthy weight is to balance energy intake and expenditure. Balancing energy intake and expenditure means that the calories consumed through food and beverages should be balanced with the calories burned through physical activity. A healthy diet rich in fruits, vegetables, whole grains, and lean proteins can help maintain weight. Regular physical activity, such as brisk walking, running, or strength training, can help maintain a healthy weight. In addition to the physical benefits, maintaining a healthy weight can also have mental and emotional benefits. It can improve self-esteem and body image and reduce the risk of developing conditions such as depression and anxiety. However, it is important to note that maintaining a healthy weight is not just about appearance. It is about overall health and well-being. A person can be at a healthy weight and still have unhealthy habits, such as not exercising regularly or consuming an unhealthy diet. On the other hand, a person may not be at a traditional "healthy" weight but still have healthy habits and a healthy body.

Focusing on overall health and well-being is important, rather than just a number on the scale. It includes following a healthy diet, regular physical activity, and stress management.

Individuals can significantly reduce their risk of developing serious health conditions and improve their quality of life by making healthy choices and maintaining a healthy weight.

CHAPTER ONE: UNDERSTANDING WEIGHT LOSS

Weight loss is losing body weight by burning more calories than are consumed. Through a combination of diet and exercise, anyone can achieve weight loss. When the body is in a calorie deficit, it uses stored fat as energy, leading to weight loss. Many factors, such as genetics, hormone imbalances, and certain medical conditions, can influence weight loss. Speaking with a healthcare professional for personalized advice on maintaining a healthy weight is important.

It is important to be mindful of the types of foods and beverages consumed and portion sizes. Healthy food choices and regular physical activity can help support weight loss and maintenance. It is also important to be patient and consistent regarding weight loss. Weight loss can take time, and focusing on healthy lifestyle changes is important rather than just trying to lose weight quickly.

How the body gains and loses weight

The body gains weight when the amount of calories consumed

through food and beverages is greater than the number of calories burned through physical activity and normal bodily functions. These excess calories are stored in the body as fat. Calories are energy found in the foods and beverages we consume. The body needs a certain amount of calories to function properly, but if we consume more calories than our body needs, the excess calories are stored in the body as fat. This can lead to weight gain over time.

On the other hand, the body loses weight when the amount of calories burned is greater than the number of calories consumed. This creates a calorie deficit, which can be achieved through diet and exercise. When the body is in a calorie deficit, it uses stored fat as energy, leading to weight loss. Physical activity plays a key role in weight loss and maintenance. Exercise helps to increase the number of calories burned by the body, which can help create a calorie deficit. In addition to burning calories, exercise has several other health benefits, such as improving heart health, strengthening bones and muscles, and reducing stress.

Diet also plays a role in weight gain and loss. A healthy diet rich in fruits, vegetables, whole grains, and lean proteins can help support weight loss and maintenance. Limiting the intake of processed foods, sugary drinks, and unhealthy fats can also help achieve and maintain a healthy weight. It is important to note that weight gain and loss are not always solely determined by diet and exercise. Several other factors, such as genetics, hormone imbalances, and certain medical conditions, can influence weight. For example, some medical conditions, such as hypothyroidism or polycystic ovary syndrome, can cause weight gain or make it more difficult to lose weight. Maintaining a healthy weight is important for overall health and well-being. It can help reduce the risk of developing serious health conditions such as obesity, type 2 diabetes, heart disease, and certain types of cancer. If you are concerned about your weight, you must speak with a healthcare professional for personalized advice and guidance.

Setting weight loss goals

Setting weight loss goals can be an effective way to help achieve and maintain a healthy weight. These are some of the tips for setting weight loss goals:

Make your goals specific and measurable: Instead of saying, "I want to lose weight," try setting a specific goal, such as "I want to lose 10 pounds in the next three months." This way, you have a clear target to work towards and can track your progress.

Set realistic goals: It is important to be realistic when setting weight loss goals. Losing 1-2 pounds per week is a safe and realistic goal. Setting unrealistic goals can lead to frustration and disappointment if they are not achieved.

Create a plan to reach your goals: Breaking your goals down into smaller, achievable steps can make them feel more manageable. For example, if your goal is to lose 10 pounds in three months, your plan might include exercising for 30 minutes each day and reducing your daily calorie intake by 500 calories.

Keep track of your progress: Tracking your progress can help you stay motivated and on track to reach your goals. Consider keeping a food diary or a fitness tracker to help monitor your progress.

Celebrate your achievements: Celebrating your successes along the way is important, no matter how small. This can help keep you motivated and encourage you to continue working towards your goals. It is important to be patient and kind to yourself as you work towards your weight loss goals. Weight loss can take time, and focusing on healthy lifestyle changes is important rather than just trying to lose weight quickly. Setting weight loss goals can be an effective way to help achieve and maintain a healthy weight.

The role of diet and exercise
in weight loss

Diet and exercise are important factors in weight loss and maintenance. Combined, they can help create a calorie deficit necessary for weight loss. Diet plays a significant role in weight loss. A healthy diet rich in fruits, vegetables, whole grains, and lean proteins can help support weight loss and maintenance. Limiting the intake of processed foods, sugary drinks, and unhealthy fats can also help achieve and maintain a healthy weight. In addition to making healthy food choices, it is also important to pay attention to portion sizes. Consuming large portions can lead to weight gain, even if the foods consumed are otherwise healthy. Exercise is another important factor in weight loss. Physical activity helps to increase the number of calories burned by the body, which can help create a calorie deficit. In addition to burning calories, exercise has several other health benefits, such as improving heart health, strengthening bones and muscles, and reducing stress. Many different types of exercise can be helpful for weight loss, such as cardio (e.g., walking, running, cycling), strength training (e.g., lifting weights), and flexibility training (e.g., yoga, Pilates). It is important to choose activities that you enjoy and fit your lifestyle, as this can make it more likely that you will stick with your exercise routine.
It is important to find a balance between diet and exercise. While exercise is important for weight loss and overall health, it is not a substitute for a healthy diet. Similarly, more than a healthy diet is needed to achieve weight loss if physical activity is not part of the equation. Combining a healthy diet with regular exercise is the most effective way to achieve and maintain a healthy weight. It is important to remember that weight loss is not a one-size-fits-all process. What works for one person may only work for one

person. Finding a balance that works for you and is sustainable in the long term is important. This may require trial and error and involve working with a healthcare professional or a registered dietitian.

Understand common myths about weight loss

There are many myths and misconceptions surrounding weight loss. These are some of the common myths:

Myth: Starving yourself is an effective way to lose weight.
Fact: While it may seem counterintuitive, drastically reducing calorie intake can slow weight loss and make it more difficult to maintain weight loss in the long term. When the body is not getting enough calories, it may go into "starvation mode" and begin to hold onto stored fat to conserve energy. This can make it more difficult to lose weight and can also lead to nutrient deficiencies.

Myth: Eating fat makes you fat.
Fact: Not all fats are created equal. While it is true that some types of fat, such as trans fats and saturated fats, can be unhealthy and contribute to weight gain, other types of fat, such as unsaturated fats, can be beneficial for weight loss. These fat types can help reduce inflammation, lower cholesterol levels, and provide essential nutrients.

Myth: Carbs are the enemy when it comes to weight loss.
Fact: Carbs are an important source of energy for the body. While it is true that some types of carbs, such as refined carbs (e.g., white bread, pasta), can be less healthy and contribute to weight gain, other types of carbs, such as complex carbs (e.g., whole grains, vegetables) can be a part of a healthy diet and support weight loss.

Myth: You have to exercise for hours a day to lose weight.
Fact: While exercise is an important part of a healthy lifestyle, it is not necessary to spend hours at the gym to see results. Research has shown that short bursts of high-intensity interval training (HIIT) can be as effective for weight loss as longer, steady-state workouts.

Myth: Weight loss supplements and "quick-fix" diets are effective for long-term weight loss.
Fact: Weight loss supplements and "quick-fix" diets are often marketed as a way to lose weight quickly and easily. However, these types of approaches are not sustainable in the long term and do not promote healthy, lasting weight loss. In addition, some weight loss supplements can have negative and harmful side effects.

It is important to be wary of these types of myths and to be critical of the information you receive about weight loss. It is always a good idea to speak with a healthcare professional or a registered dietitian for personalized, evidence-based advice on maintaining a healthy weight.

CHAPTER TWO: DEVELOPING A WEIGHT LOSS PLAN

There are many potential benefits to developing a weight loss plan. Some people may want to lose weight to improve their overall health and reduce their risk of developing heart disease, diabetes, and high blood pressure. Others may want to lose weight to improve their appearance or self-esteem. A weight loss plan can help you to set specific goals and track your progress, which can be motivating. It can also provide structure and accountability, helping you to stay on track and make healthy choices. Developing a weight loss plan can also help you to make sustainable lifestyle changes, rather than trying fad diets or quick fixes that may not be effective in the long term.

Assessing your current eating habits

To assess your current eating habits for weight loss, you can start by keeping a food diary for a few days or a week. In your food diary, record everything you eat and drink, the time of day, and any accompanying circumstances (such as feeling stressed or tired). Be as detailed as possible, including portion sizes and any condiments or seasonings you use.

Next, review your food diary and look for patterns or areas where you can make changes. Some questions to consider might include the following:

Do you eat regular, balanced meals, skip meals or eat irregularly?

Do you eat various fruits, vegetables, and other nutrient-dense foods or rely heavily on processed or fast foods?

Do you drink enough water and limit your intake of sugary drinks?

Do you eat when you are hungry or for reasons such as boredom, stress, or emotional comfort?

Based on your food diary and your answers to these questions, you can identify specific changes you can make to your eating habits to support your weight loss goals. It may be helpful to work with a healthcare professional or a registered dietitian to develop a personalized plan.

Creating a calorie deficit

To create a calorie deficit, you need to burn more calories than you consume. There are a few different ways to do this:

Reduce your calorie intake: This can be done by making healthier food choices, such as choosing lean proteins, whole grains, and plenty of fruits and vegetables, and cutting out added sugars and unhealthy fats. You can also try using smaller plates and bowls to help you eat smaller portions.

Increase your physical activity: Regular exercise can help burn more calories and create a calorie deficit. Aim for at least 150 minutes of moderate-intensity activity, such as brisk walking or cycling, or 75 minutes of vigorous-intensity activity, such as running or high-intensity interval training, per week.

Combine both strategies: It is generally most effective to reduce your calorie intake and increase your physical activity for maximum weight loss. This can help you create a larger calorie deficit and lose weight more quickly.

It is important to note that everyone's calorie needs are different based on age, gender, weight, height, and activity level. It can be helpful to work with a healthcare professional or registered dietitian to determine your specific calorie needs and create a safe and effective plan for you.

Choosing healthy foods and snacks
There are many different types of healthy foods and snacks that you can incorporate into your weight loss plan. Some options to consider might include the following:

Fruits and vegetables are rich in nutrients and low in calories, making them a great choice for weight loss. Choose a variety of colorful fruits and vegetables to ensure you get a wide range of nutrients.

Lean proteins: Foods like chicken, turkey, fish, beans, and tofu are high in protein and can help you feel full and satisfied. They can also help to preserve muscle mass during weight loss.

Whole grains: Choose whole grain bread, cereals, rice, and pasta over refined grains, as they are higher in fiber and nutrients.

Nuts and seeds: These are high in healthy fats, protein, and fiber and can help to keep you feeling full and satisfied. Just be sure to watch your portion sizes, which are also high in calories.

Healthy fats: Foods like avocados, olive oil, and nuts are high in healthy fats and can help to keep you feeling full and satisfied. Just be sure to watch your portion sizes, which are also high in calories.

Low-fat dairy: Dairy products like milk, yogurt, and cheese are rich in protein and calcium, but be sure to choose low-fat or non-fat options to cut down on calories and unhealthy fats.

When choosing snacks, look for options that are nutrient-dense and low in calories. Some healthy snack ideas might include fruit, vegetables with hummus or guacamole, nuts, or low-fat yogurt.

Incorporating physical activity into your routine

To incorporate physical activity into your routine, try finding activities you enjoy, such as walking, running, swimming, cycling, or dancing. Make a schedule and set aside specific times for exercise. If you are new to exercise or haven't been active, start with small amounts of activity and gradually increase your duration and intensity over time. Mix your activities to challenge your body, including strength training, yoga, and cardio workouts. Consider finding a workout partner or joining a fitness class to stay motivated and accountable. You can also incorporate physical activity into your daily routine by taking the stairs instead of the elevator, walking during lunch breaks, or biking to work. Remember to listen to your body and avoid overdoing it. Warm up before the activity, cool down afterward, and stop if you feel pain or discomfort. If you have any health concerns, you should talk to a healthcare professional before starting a new exercise program.

Seeking support from friends and family

Seeking support from friends and family can be a helpful way to stay motivated and accountable during your weight loss journey. Here are a few ways to involve your loved ones in your efforts:

Share your goals: Let your friends and family know what you are trying to achieve, and ask for their support.

Find a workout buddy: Having someone to exercise with can make it more fun and help to keep you motivated.

Ask for help with meal planning and preparation: Involve your friends and family in choosing healthy meals and snacks, and ask for their help with meal prep.

Share your progress: Keep your loved ones updated and ask for their encouragement and support.

Celebrate your successes: When you reach a goal or make progress, celebrate with your friends and family. This can help to keep you motivated and show them how much their support means to you.

It's important to remember that everyone is different, and what works for one person may not work for another. Be open to trying different approaches and finding what works best for you. If you need additional support or guidance, consider seeking the help of a healthcare professional or a registered dietitian.

CHAPTER THREE: OVERCOMING CHALLENGES

Emotional eating is the practice of using food as a way to cope with negative emotions, such as stress, boredom, or sadness. It can be a common challenge for people trying to lose weight, leading to overeating and making it difficult to stick to a healthy diet. If you struggle with emotional eating, there are a few strategies that may help prevent being overweight:

Identify your triggers: The first step in managing emotional eating is identifying what emotions or situations tend to trigger it. This can help you become more aware of your patterns and find ways to cope with your emotions healthily.

Find alternative coping mechanisms: Instead of turning to food, try finding other ways to cope with negative emotions. This can include exercise, meditation, or talking to a friend or therapist. Exercise can be particularly helpful, as it can help to reduce stress and improve your mood.

Practice mindful eating: When you eat, try to be present and fully engage in the experience. Pay attention to your food, savor the flavors and textures, and eat slowly. This can help you be more aware of your hunger and fullness cues and make it easier to stop eating when satisfied.

Seek support: Talk to a friend, family member, or therapist about your struggles with emotional eating. They can provide emotional support and help you to develop healthy coping strategies. It can also be helpful to join a support group or seek the help of a healthcare professional or registered dietitian.

Set realistic goals: Try to keep everything the same. Instead, focus on making small, manageable changes to your diet and lifestyle. Set achievable goals and celebrate your successes along the way.

Practice self-care: Take care of your physical and emotional needs. Get enough sleep, practice stress management techniques, and find activities that bring you joy and relaxation.

Emotional eating is a common challenge; it is important to be kind to yourself and remember that change takes time. With practice and support, you can learn to manage your emotions healthily and break the cycle of emotional eating.

Handling setbacks and plateaus

Setbacks and plateaus are a normal part of the weight loss journey, and it is important to remember that progress may not always be linear. It can be easy to get discouraged when you hit a plateau or experience a setback, but it is important to stay positive and keep going. Here are a few strategies for handling setbacks and plateaus:

One thing you can do is reflect on your progress so far. Take a step back and look at the changes you have made and the progress you have achieved. It can be helpful to keep track of your progress by regularly weighing yourself and measuring your waist circumference. Seeing your progress can help keep you motivated and remind you that you are making progress, even if it is not as fast as you would like. Another strategy is to reassess your diet and exercise plan. If you have hit a plateau, it may be helpful to review your plan to see if there are any changes you can make. This can include increasing your physical activity or changing your workouts to challenge your body in new ways. It can also be helpful to seek the help of a registered dietitian to review your diet and ensure you are getting the nutrients you need. It is also important to have a healthy relationship with food and to allow yourself to enjoy treats in moderation. You may be more likely to fall off track if you are too restrictive. Allowing yourself to indulge occasionally can help to prevent feelings of deprivation and make it easier to stick to your plan overall. Feel free to seek support if you are feeling overwhelmed or discouraged. Talk to a friend, family member, or healthcare professional for encouragement and help.

Staying motivated

Staying motivated can be a challenge regarding weight loss, but it is an important factor in achieving your goals. To stay motivated, try setting specific, achievable goals for yourself, such as losing a certain number of pounds or inches or exercising a certain number of times per week. Keeping track of your progress can also be a great source of motivation, so regularly weigh yourself, measure your waist circumference, and celebrate your successes. Having a support system of friends, family, or a support group can also help you stay motivated. They can provide encouragement and accountability and help you stay on track. Remember to stay positive, that weight loss is a journey, and it is normal to have setbacks and plateaus. Reward yourself when you reach a goal or make progress to stay motivated and celebrate your achievements. Finally, trying different strategies and finding what works best for you to stay motivated on your weight loss journey is important.

CHAPTER FOUR: MAINTENANCE AND LONG-TERM SUCCESS

As you get closer to your weight loss goals, you may need to phase out your weight loss plan gradually. This can be challenging, but it is an important step in maintaining weight loss and developing a healthy, sustainable lifestyle. Here are a few tips for phasing out your weight loss plan:

Gradually increase your calorie intake: As you lose weight, your body's energy needs will decrease. It is important to gradually increase your calorie intake to match your new needs rather than drastically increasing it all at once.

Continue to focus on healthy eating: While it is okay to indulge occasionally, it is important to continue to focus on eating a healthy, balanced diet. This can include a variety of fruits, vegetables, whole grains, lean proteins, and healthy fats.

Keep up with physical activity: Regular physical activity is important for maintaining weight loss and overall health. Aim to incorporate various activities into your routine, and continue to challenge yourself to improve your fitness level.

Find a balance: It is important to balance structure and flexibility in your eating and exercise habits. This can help to prevent feelings of deprivation and make it easier to stick to a healthy lifestyle long-term.

Seek support: If you need help in phasing out your weight loss plan, consider seeking the support of a healthcare professional or registered dietitian. They can guide and help you develop a plan that works for you.

Staying active and maintaining a healthy diet

Staying active and maintaining a healthy diet is important for overall physical and mental well-being. Regular physical activity can help to improve cardiovascular health, increase strength and flexibility, and reduce the risk of developing certain chronic conditions such as obesity, type 2 diabetes, and heart disease. A healthy diet, on the other hand, can help provide the nutrients and energy needed to support a physically active lifestyle and promote overall health and well-being. To stay active, it is important to incorporate various activities into your routine, such as walking, jogging, cycling, swimming, or playing sports. It is generally recommended to aim for at least 150 minutes of moderate-intensity activity per week or 75 minutes of vigorous-intensity activity.

Regarding diet, it is important to focus on consuming various nutrient-dense foods, including fruits, vegetables, whole grains, lean proteins, and healthy fats. It is also important to limit the intake of added sugars, sodium, and unhealthy fats. Maintaining a healthy diet and being physically active can help support a healthy weight and contribute to improved mood, increased energy levels, and better sleep.

Dealing with weight regain

Dealing with weight regain can be a challenging and frustrating experience. If you have recently regained weight after successfully losing it, it is important to remember that it is common for weight to fluctuate, and it does not necessarily mean that you have failed. Several factors can contribute to weight regain, such as changes in lifestyle, stress, medical conditions, or medication. To effectively deal with weight regain, it is important to identify and address the underlying cause. This may involve changing your diet, increasing physical activity, managing stress, or seeking support from a healthcare professional. It is also important to remember to be kind to yourself and focus on your progress rather than any setbacks. Instead of getting discouraged, try to use the experience as an opportunity to learn and make adjustments as needed. It may be helpful to set small, achievable goals and to seek support from friends, family, or a healthcare professional. Remember that the journey towards a healthy weight is not always a straight line and that it is normal to encounter challenges along the way.

CONCLUSION

"The Weight Loss Journey: A Step-by-Step Guide to Success" has provided a comprehensive and practical approach to achieving and maintaining a healthy weight. Through evidence-based strategies and a focus on sustainability, this book has equipped readers with the tools and knowledge needed to create a personalized weight loss plan that works for them. By following the steps outlined in this book, readers have the potential to not only lose weight but also to improve their overall health and well-being. The journey towards a healthy weight is not always easy, but by taking it one step at a time and staying committed to your goals, you can successfully navigate the challenges and reach your destination. Remember to be kind to yourself, celebrate your progress, and seek support when needed. With determination and a positive attitude, you can create a healthier and happier future for yourself.

ABOUT THE AUTHOR

Steven Smith

Steven Smith holds a doctorate in Construction Management. He has published several research articles locally and internationally.

BOOKS BY THIS AUTHOR

The Dictionary Of Construction Teminologies: A Compendium Of Knowledge For Students, Academics, Practitioners And House Owners

The dictionary of construction terminologies book is a comprehensive reference guide that provides definitions and explanations of the technical language and jargon used in the construction industry. It is an invaluable resource for professionals working in construction, as well as for students learning about the industry or for individuals looking to understand construction-related concepts better.

The Wealth Creators' Manual: A Handbook For Financial Success

The Wealth Creators' Manual is a comprehensive guide to financial success. This handbook offers practical strategies and techniques for building wealth and achieving financial stability. Inside, you'll find expert advice on budgeting, saving, investing, and building passive income streams. With a focus on long-term planning and smart decision-making, this manual is an essential resource for anyone looking to take control of their financial future. Whether you're just starting out on your wealth creation journey or looking to fine-tune your existing financial plan, The Wealth Creators' Manual has something for everyone. With its clear, concise writing and actionable tips, this book is a must-read for anyone looking to secure their financial future.